Doctor Robert Lefever

The Promis Recovery Centre

GW00357299

*for Elizabeth
with good wishes
Robert*

healing

PROMIS

The PROMIS Primer

Written by Dr Robert Lefever

PROMIS Recovery Centre Limited
The Old Court House, Pinners Hill
Nonington, Nr. Canterbury
Kent CT15 4LL. UK
www.promis.co.uk

© Dr Robert Lefever 2002

ISBN 1 871013 18 6

Design and production by Rainbow, Ipswich IP5 3RY, England.
Printed in Basauri, Spain by Grafo SA.

**To
my son Henry
in admiration
and with love**

Contents

Acknowledgements

To Sarah Oaten for typing the manuscript,

to Dr. Harriet Harvey-Wood for editing it,

to my teachers and patients - often one and the same.

Chapter One

Treatment and Healing

Treatment and healing are not the same thing. Treatment is what doctors and nurses and other professional helpers do. Healing is something that happens in the individual body or mind of the patient.

Two people with the identical condition may be given the same treatment and yet one is healed and the other is not. They differ in how they respond. Sometimes the reason for an individual response is physical. No two people are exactly alike and the same disease will inevitably affect them slightly differently. For example, the physical structure of the heart and arteries of some people may make them particularly vulnerable to cardio-vascular disease. Some are born with kinks in the coronary arteries or with a tendency towards having a high cholesterol level in the blood but others have no such problems. Correspondingly two people may both have diabetes by name but in fact have two very different medical conditions although both are called diabetes simply because of a raised blood sugar. The one patient may be young and require Insulin and the other may be older and require no treatment other than careful dietary management. Two people may both be exposed to the bacterium that causes tuberculosis. One develops a terrible disease whereas the other shrugs it off and the only evidence that he or she has ever had it is a small calcified area in the top of one lung. Two people may suffer identical injuries, such as a fractured hip in old age. One will get better but the other will be permanently crippled and may die. Two people may be divorced or bereaved. One will somehow make a new life but the other may remain permanently scarred.

Healing depends very much on the individual make-up of patients both physically and emotionally. Obviously it also depends on social, cultural and economic factors. Rich people have more resources and it is often true that money can indeed make a significant difference to healthcare. There are occasions when people have more money than sense but it is generally true in the world at large that poverty is the greatest cause of ill health. Yet even two people who are equally rich or another two people who are equally poor will have a different capacity for healing. One may do well and the other very badly. Two people given identical treatments will react very differently. One person may get over an operation very quickly whereas another may take a long time to get back to normal physical, mental, emotional and social function.

Healing is therefore very much an individual process as far as each and every patient is concerned. Doctors, nurses and other professional or personal helpers play their part and economic and social conditions are a major influence but even then it is the individual response of the patient that makes a crucial difference.

Body and mind work together to such an extent that they should really be seen as one unit: body/mind. When we are ill we become depressed and we find it difficult to think straight. When we are depressed we are more prone to physical illness. None the less some conditions are more specifically physical and others more specifically mental. For example, a fractured finger is almost exclusively physical and schizophrenia is almost exclusively mental. Someone who has a fractured finger is unlikely to develop a severe mental illness as a complication of that fracture. Even a concert pianist would be depressed and anxious rather than mentally ill as such. Correspondingly, someone who has a mental illness such as schizophrenia is not directly more likely to fracture a finger. An episode of violence could result in a fractured finger but that could happen to anybody. None the less most clinical conditions are not as clear-cut as these two extremes. People who have been recently bereaved have a high mortality risk: they have an increased risk of dying in the early months after being bereaved in comparison with other people of the same age and general health. Influenza is a major killing disease: more people died of the influenza pandemic at the time of the First World War than died in the hostilities. Yet influenza and other viral infections do not simply affect the body. They also affect the way that people feel. Some individuals go on to get a post-viral depressive illness and we really do not know why these people should be more prone than others to this particular complication.

Certainly some people appear to be more emotionally as well as physically resilient than others. They are sometimes said to have more "moral fibre" (whatever that may be). They may almost shrug off severe illnesses or accidents. They may be determined to prove how quickly they can get well - and they do. Others may be laid low by a much lesser physical or emotional trauma. They may sometimes be described as "weak-willed" or even "pathetic". Yet is this difference in resilience really something that an individual can control? Were the strong ones born with that capacity? Or were they lucky in not previously experiencing significant emotional or physical trauma that might have made them more vulnerable?

We tend to be very critical of people who "make a fuss". We may not see this as an "illness" in its own right. We become exasperated with their moans and groans and their apparent incapacity to do even the most straightforward things to help themselves. Yet this "dis-ease" might be seen as a "disease" that particularly affects some people. Why should this be so? Are they just trying to get a free ride on the productive work of the rest of the population? Are they so wrapped up in their own concerns that they never consider anybody else? Do they need nothing more than "a kick up the arse"? Or are they unwell in a particular way that leads them to particular misery that is compounded by social rejection when other people get fed-up with them?

Certainly, telling these people to "pull themselves together" does not work. Very often it is not simply that they won't but that they can't. To say "of course they can" completely under-estimates the problem. It is like telling an alcoholic to stop drinking. That is perfectly sensible advice but the alcoholic would not be alcoholic if he or she could follow that advice. To be sure, the wimps and misfits and walking disasters of this world are exasperating and, to be sure, they would benefit a great deal from learning to take more responsibility for themselves and becoming less dependent upon other people. However, the interesting question is how these people came to be like that. They collect an enormous amount of physical, emotional, mental and social pathology - far more than their fair share. Were they made like that or did they suffer some particular trauma in childhood or in later life that made them more prone to illness and dis-ease of one kind or another? Why do they seem not to learn from experience? Why are they always in trouble with one thing or another? Why do they heal so badly after physical or emotional stresses?

Come to that, are we ourselves perfect? Are there not some things that still worry us years or even decades after the initial trauma? Why are we still unable to forget those things and simply move on? What is it that keeps us stuck? Why is it that some mannerisms, attitudes and prejudices that may have sprung from particular incidents have in time become so ingrained into our natures that they become features of our personalities? Why can't we "shake ourselves out of it"? Are we really all that different in this respect from life's misfits? How much do we fit? We may earn our livings and pay our rent and support our families but have we really healed from the emotional stresses and strains of earlier experiences? Have we fully got over the traumas of our childhood and earlier adult life? Have we recovered from the hurts and unfairnesses that we have endured? Or are we still damaged in one way or another, however stable we may appear to be to others and however determined we are to give that impression? Are we ourselves healed or have we merely survived? When we consider all our assets, have we really been anything more than lucky, in one way or another, in comparison with other people?

For example, intelligence is a natural gift and we can take no credit for that. Furthermore, what we do with our native intelligence may be largely a question of response to opportunity. In the last analysis there may be relatively little that is truly to our own credit. We may have worked hard and taken difficult decisions and made various sacrifices - but, given our natural abilities and social opportunities, should anything less have been expected of us?

If we do heal well, relative to other people, it may equally be because we have been lucky. We may have natural gifts of that nature. We may have suffered fewer traumatic experiences and these may have been of lesser severity than those of other people. We may like to consider that we are "winners" but it may be more true that we have been lucky. We might with advantage look at other people with more understanding and compassion when we come to see how truly lucky we ourselves have been.

Those of us who are in the "helping" professions may sometimes like to think of ourselves as "healers". This is a very dangerous concept. We may become arrogant and even uncaring as a result of believing that we have special qualities. We may come to expect the appreciation of others over and above the payment of our salaries. We may seek not only thanks but admiration and even adulation. At worst, we may want to be worshipped rather than simply given credit for our technical competence. When we consider ourselves to be especially virtuous we may actually become very damaging to those who ask for our help. We become harmers rather than healers. We become sloppy, inefficient and un-caring precisely because we rate ourselves so highly. In truth we have every right to give ourselves credit for our practiced technical skills - but so has a plumber or tennis player or secretary or housewife or anyone else. There should be nothing extra-ordinary about the "helping" professions. If we see ourselves as "healers" rather than technicians we risk causing ourselves and our patients great damage. A surgeon is a surgeon, not a healer. A nurse is a nurse, not a healer. A psychiatrist is a psychiatrist, not a healer. Each has his or her skills to offer - and, hopefully, can at the same time be polite and considerate, caring and nurturing. Yet there are many other people who also have the capacity to be polite and considerate, caring and nurturing: these are personal attributes rather than technical qualifications. Furthermore, some non-medical people seem to possess amazing powers of "healing": we feel "better" in their presence and there may be some technical procedure - such as dowsing or the laying-on of hands, that may have a healing effect that currently has no scientific explanation. The "placebo" effect in which people will believe what they want to believe, may not be the full answer. Some non-medical people seem to have "the gift of healing". Many professional helpers may lack it.

Treatment and healing are not the same thing at all.

Chapter Two

Helping

I have done a total of something in the region of a quarter of a million consultations in my life as a family doctor. As a general medical practitioner I have more of an interest in people than in specific illnesses or clinical conditions. Obviously I have to be familiar with a wide range of clinical conditions because that is precisely why patients come to see me: they want to tap into my technical knowledge. They want to get a precise diagnosis and appropriate treatment. However, any working doctor knows that clinical practice is not as straightforward as that. There are often multiple diagnoses covering a range of physical, mental, emotional and social aspects of the patient's life and hence there may be a range of "treatments" - if, that is, one decides to treat at all and if the patient considers it appropriate for us to do so. Quite often a patient and I may have very different perspectives on what might be really important. For example, a patient may be absolutely convinced that a particular physical symptom has a physical cause whereas I may believe the true cause to be psychological or social. At other times, another patient might believe that a particular symptom is trivial whereas I would know from my technical training that it could be very significant indeed.

Recently a patient was referred to me by a consultant cardiologist who had given up on trying to reassure this man that he had no heart disease whatever. One test after another was negative and the cardiologist did not consider it responsible to go on doing further physical tests to find the cause of the sensations of tightness in the chest and tinglings in the arms. In due course, from the broader perspective of general practice, I learnt that the patient is secretly homosexual and is terrified that his episodes of anonymous promiscuity might have lead to AIDS or hepatitis B or C or other debilitating conditions. His fear did indeed give him palpitations. Yet he still refuses to accept my explanation. Far from being healed by my explanation, he is irritated by it. He wants me to send him to another cardiologist or a neurologist. He asked me for a copy of all his records so that he could take them to further specialists and I anticipate that he may well decide not to see me again.

Another patient whom I saw on the same day complained of feeling a bit wobbly and dizzy and nauseous. He also complained of tingling sensations in the left side of his tongue and face and in the left fourth and fifth fingers and in the left big toe. He found these symptoms a bit strange but was not really worried about them. I was. I arranged for an immediate MRI scan of the brain and for subsequent emergency admission to a neurology unit when the report of the MRI scan showed an inflammatory area in the medulla at the base of the brain.

In both these cases I relied primarily upon a "sixth" sense. Inevitably a quarter of a million consultations gives me an immense clinical experience. I have seen conditions like these before and I have learnt - often from previous mistakes - to make a judgement on whether the patient is "ill" or not and what type of treatment might be appropriate. In my view the first patient has an illness no less severe than the second. He has a significant mortality risk through suicide and I shall certainly follow him up if he allows me to do so. The second probably has disseminated sclerosis and the severity of this initial attack may not necessarily imply that the future progression of his illness will be equally dramatic. The first patient may well die before the second and, in the remaining years that each has to live, the first patient may have a much more wretched time than the second.

At present there is no guarantee of a cure for either patient: in neither case can I tell them that they will be healed. Reassuring the first patient that he does not have heart disease and that there is a perfectly reasonable emotional explanation for his symptoms does not necessarily heal him at all. He may well stick to his own perception regardless of however carefully and sensitively I may try to approach him. The second patient may well come back to me asking for my opinion on treatment with Interferon or even with cannabis but he will know as well as I do that these are treatments - of a kind - rather than cures.

The first patient has a disorder of perception whereas the second will probably understand very well precisely what he has got. Of the two, the disorder of perception is in many ways more devastating. Why should a patient seek treatment for a condition that he does not believe he has got in the first place? Why should he trust a doctor who does not agree with what he considers to be the obvious cause of his symptoms? The second patient has every reason to be frightened - and so does his wife. Their whole lives will be turned upside down by this diagnosis and by the implications for his employment and for their life together, particularly as his wife is currently pregnant with their first child. Yet still it is the first patient who in some ways gives me greater concern: the second patient, with disseminated sclerosis, will probably find a way of living within the constraints imposed by his illness whereas the first patient may well continue to be tortured until he ultimately destroys himself. To give the first patient antidepressants or tranquillisers - so that I could say at his inquest that I had "done everything I could to help him" would simply be a cop out. I don't believe that those drugs ever really help anyone whereas they are often very damaging. They do not help people to solve problems and they are often used in overdose by people who commit suicide. Nonetheless, there is a chance - through appropriate psychotherapy - that this first patient could be healed of his affliction whereas there is currently no chance for the second other than through spontaneous remission which does happen occasionally.

In general medical practice it is my job to do the best I can for the patient sitting in front of me. In the case of the patient with disseminated sclerosis, the best I could do was to get a rapid diagnosis and referral. From now on all I have to offer is human comfort - and I don't belittle that. For the first patient, with the anxiety state, I do not believe that a consultant psychiatrist would have any more to offer than I should be able to offer myself. Indeed, this type of problem should really be my speciality precisely because I work in the community. I should be familiar with the general stresses and strains of the "normal" population whereas hospital doctors may sometimes get isolated in their ivory towers, seeing pathology rather than people.

From the vantage point of general medical practice, I have become increasingly aware of my responsibility towards patients who do not have the clinical conditions that I was trained to recognise during my under-graduate years in teaching hospital as well as those who do. I have some patients - three to be precise - whom I have looked after as their general medical practitioner for over thirty years. We are part of each other's lives by now. Another patient whom I met last week for the first time, is already an important part of my life because her story of forced ingestion of a drug and subsequent rape in a public lavatory, would affect anyone - or certainly should, I hope, bring out the best in any doctor (although the police surgeon she met seems to have been rather unimpressive). In between these extremes of time, the majority of my patients, as with any other doctor, keep coming back to see me because they consider me to be "their" doctor. They trust me to give them personalised care: to be on their side and to understand their perspectives as well as simply to give them appropriate physical treatments. In the course of a day I may give them whatever treatment may be appropriate for an acute medical condition. In the course of a year my nurse practitioner monitors them for conditions, such as raised blood pressure or diabetes or abnormalities on cervical smear tests and other conditions that may require regular monitoring even though the patient may have no symptoms. In the course of a decade or more I become aware of the long-term effects of physical or emotional trauma. I see how someone's childhood experience or divorce or bereavement or road accident or acute illness has long-term knock-on effects.

It was largely as a result of this long-term perspective that I developed an interest in addictive disease. Alcoholism, drug addiction, eating disorders and other compulsive behaviours lead to immense damage not only in the individual but also in his or her family and place of work and in society at large. Here is a field of primary responsibility for general medical practitioners. By and large all that hospital doctors have to offer in this area of clinical practice is emergency treatments for accidents or overdoses or other disasters but then the patient is often returned to the general practitioner with a letter saying that the patient has been advised to change his or her behaviour. The general practitioner, however, has seen the patient progressively deteriorate over the years despite all manner of good advice and any number of information sheets on the dangers of this or that particular substance or behaviour. Of course, the general practitioner can simply shrug and say "This is not real medical practice: this is not what I was trained to do". By contrast, in my own case I believe that it was my training that was wrong. It should have been what I was trained to do.

I was trained largely in clinical conditions that I would see in hospital - but, along with half of my professional colleagues, I am not a hospital doctor. Last week I went to a detailed postgraduate lecture on Crohn's disease and learnt, among other things, that I should see seven new cases a year for every one hundred thousand patients. I calculated that I should therefore see one new case every seven years. Why on earth would I ever want to know anything about Crohn's disease other than to know how to diagnose it and refer the patient on to a hospital doctor? On the other hand, I see people with emotional problems every day of my life. Up to one third of all consultations in general medical practice are with people whose primary problem is emotional rather than physical - and yet I had absolutely no training whatever in medical school on how to deal with these problems as opposed to major psychiatric illness.

As with other medical students, I was taught how to prescribe antidepressants or tranquillisers or sleeping tablets - and the end result of that teaching is that one third of the adult population is prescribed these drugs on a regular basis. That is an immense indictment of our training in medical school. It is absolutely appalling that we should treat people in this way and even support our "treatment" by inventing diagnoses such as "clinical depression", "agitated depression", "personality disorder" and other spurious medical conditions in which the diagnosis serves primarily to separate the normal population (doctors) from the pathological (patients). We con ourselves into believing that we are helping - or even healing - when in fact we may be pontificating and poisoning. These may seem harsh words but the analysis of doctors' prescribing habits speaks for itself at a time when our knowledge of brain biochemistry is still in its infancy.

I do not blame the pharmaceutical industry. They do their job in researching new drugs that they hope will be helpful. Understandably they advertise their products and they promote them in any way they can. That is part of their commercial business and I should rather have a free market in which the pharmaceutical industry researches and tests than a State controlled service that produced nothing new of any value and that ultimately regiments not only treatment but also diagnosis, even to the extreme of determining that dissidents are mentally ill. It is doctors alone who have the responsibility for what we prescribe or do in other ways in the guise of "treatment". If we say we have insufficient time to do anything other than prescribe, we should do nothing at all.

To prescribe or take a pharmaceutical drug is a major statement in the minds of both doctor and patient. The doctor says "this is something I believe you really need" and the patient says, "I am sick, which is why I need something". These are very profound statements indeed and, when taken casually, can lead to a very great deal of damage. Far from "healing" their patients, doctors can become the source of a great deal of psycho-pathology, leaving their patients to become dependent upon "a pill for every ill" and believe that they are "sick" and that they "need" treatment, when in fact neither statement may be true.

Florence Nightingale gave the exhortation that we should first do no harm. We should certainly remember that advice today when vast numbers of patients are admitted to hospital directly as a result of something that a doctor did inappropriately or inadequately. Patients take their lives in their hands when they come to see us. We would benefit not only from a healthy dose of humility but also a healthy dose of awe for the capacity of the human body and mind to look after itself and heal itself. Perhaps the first question that any doctor should ask is "Am I necessary at all - beyond listening to the patient, making an appropriate physical examination, and then giving information?" Along with other health professionals, we may not be the helpers - let alone healers - that we think we are.

healing

14

Chapter Three

Who Guards the Guards?

In six years of university and medical school training I never once had to examine my own psyche. Nor, for that matter, was it ever examined by anyone else. I was assessed for my technical knowledge: nothing more than that. Even my practical skills were largely unassessed. In my time as a medical student no one ever saw me sew up a wound. I even delivered babies with only a midwife rather than a doctor being present, although this should be no surprise because most babies are delivered by midwives rather than by doctors. As far as my mental fitness to practise is concerned, however, I had absolutely no assessment whatever. It was assumed of all medical students that if we were clever enough to pass our written and clinical examinations we would be appropriately equipped to become doctors.

My own belief is that medical students should be selected on a far wider basis than at present. A knowledge of scientific subjects should be matched by evidence of human interests. After all, patients are human beings, not simply physiological machines. The same also applies to doctors: we get the same illnesses - mental as well as physical - as our patients. Yet it cannot be right that my mental and emotional health was never examined at all and I don't suppose that I was the exception either then or now.

I am not implying that only those students who are "perfect" physically, emotionally and mentally should qualify as doctors. We all have blemishes to some degree, some more than others. Indeed, the concept of the "wounded healer" is very important in psychological terms: sometimes those of us who have defects of one kind or another can be very empathic with, and helpful towards, patients who have similar or other defects. None the less, there must be a level at which a defect in a doctor or other professional helper becomes a major handicap and a risk to patients. It is unacceptable that there is no assessment of these risks in our student years.

Almost half the product of medical schools will finish up in general medical practice. When we remember that one third of all general practitioners' consultations are primarily emotional in content, and all consultations have some emotional factor that needs to be taken into account, it must be important for doctors in general medical practice to be able to communicate successfully with their patients on emotional matters. Doctors who themselves have emotional difficulties of one kind or another will find that particular aspect of general medical practice extremely challenging. In short, they may be ill equipped for the job that they actually have to do in practice, irrespective of what they were trained to do in medical school.

Even in hospital work there is a significant emotional component to every consultation. The patients of surgeons will often be frightened and those of physicians often confused. Those of psychiatrists may have fundamental disorders of perception - they simply do not see the world as other people see it - and they may be frightened and confused as well. Doctors hoping to heal patients in any of these areas of clinical practice will have an exceptionally difficult time if they themselves are emotionally stressed or if they are uncomfortable with the emotional, rather than simply physical, aspects of their work. Even psychiatrists may shy away from emotional rather than intellectual or chemical aspects of their work: they may prefer to analyse or prescribe rather than comfort or encourage. Doctors of all kinds may at times feel that the "human" aspects of their work are not really "medical" in so far as they were not trained to deal with this aspect of their patients' problems. With some justification, they may believe that other people might be better placed to deal with these issues. None the less, that is easier said than done: the patient has every reason to expect a doctor or other health professional to be a fully rounded personality. After all, if doctors are not at ease themselves then how could they help other people to be at ease? In practical terms, however, there may be no one else available to whom they can delegate the emotional component of a consultation and, as emphasised, every consultation has some emotional component so this aspect of a doctor's work can not be avoided altogether.

It could be argued that medical school training is already lengthy and complex and that it has to focus first of all on technical matters that are the exclusive province of health professionals. A doctor who is kind and considerate but who does not know one heart sound from another, or know how to interpret abnormal liver function tests, would be a menace. Even so, medical education that is focused almost exclusively on the technical aspects of each subject - even psychiatry - is not a rounded education and does not produce rounded doctors. Our patients deserve better than that, particularly in general medical practice where so many emotional and social factors have to be taken into account alongside the strictly physical and mental components of patients' problems.

Among my own contemporaries at medical school there were some significantly disturbed souls. One committed suicide. One got through three wives within five years of qualification. One was not simply promiscuous but should probably be diagnosed as a sex and love addict. One was definitely alcoholic. I don't know about the rest but I suspect we all have problems to some degree. I myself am a compulsive gambler and that showed itself quite clearly at the time that I was a medical student. I am also a compulsive helper, sometimes helping others primarily in order to feel good about myself. This goes beyond normal professional satisfaction and can lead to self-delusion as well as professional burn-out.

It seems to me that there are two fundamental questions:

i.   Is there a value in assessing the emotional and mental health of medical students and other health professionals as early as possible in their training?

ii.   Who should perform that evaluation and what authority should be given to the conclusions?

The answer to the first question seems obvious until we consider the second. *Quis custodes custodiet?* Who guards the guards? I remember a time when a small group of professional colleagues in general medical practice (we were each involved in the training of medical students and junior doctors) seriously suggested that I should seek psychiatric help when I forcibly disagreed with them on the subject of whether communication skills can be taught or whether, as I believe, they are primarily innate. I may be wrong on the issue but the suggestion that I should therefore need mental help strikes me as being totalitarian. Well it would appear that way to me myself, wouldn't it? Were they right? Would I see it even if they were? The issues are not as simple as they might first appear to be.

It also seems to me that there should be different levels of emotional assessment for different levels of clinical work. A researcher, an academic or a laboratory scientist should not be expected to have the same human inter-personal skills, emotional resilience and social and cultural interests as a general medical practitioner. Equally a hospital physician, surgeon or psychiatrist would need more personal maturity and communicative skill than those doctors whose work rarely brings them into contact with patients - but they might require less than those of us who work in general medical practice. For us, the personal skills are paramount - otherwise we cannot do the job.

I recall a lady doctor of middle European origin telling me passionately how much she hated her patients in general medical practice. I wonder that any of them survived her "care". I also recall the secretary and nurse of a young doctor in a group practice telling me that he had demanded that they should treat him with respect. How on earth did he come to be in his professional position without realising that respect has to be earned? If he makes fundamental inter-personal errors at that level with his staff then what on earth does he do in his consultations with patients?

Yet who am I to imply criticism of these professional colleagues? I don't know the stresses under which they work or live and I may be the last person to be able to make accurate assessment of myself. None the less, I think it reasonable to question how either of those doctors came to be working in general medical practice. Did they simply fail to become something else? Was Lord Moran, Winston Churchill's doctor, correct when he said that general practitioners are the failures of the medical profession? If so, is that safe? One need not look solely at the case of Dr Harold Shipman, the mass murderer, to be concerned about this issue. But, come to think of it, how did he get through the checks and balances on his emotional and mental health when he was in medical school or in his early - or even later - years in clinical practice? I suspect he did so because there weren't any.

Chapter Four

Who Helps the Helpers?

There is an old saying that a doctor who treats himself for his own medical problems has a fool for a physician. Patients need an impartial eye or ear if they are to get the best clinical judgement. We can never provide this for ourselves.

For physical illness this should be no great problem. Peter Baird repaired the ruptured flexor tendon on my right ring finger, John Stubbs took out my gallbladder and John Collins treated me for a lung infection due to mycoplasma. In each case I was happy to place myself in their care and they gave me excellent service.

It was a different matter altogether when I was under emotional stress. In the first place I did not believe that I had a problem: I was so wrapped up in myself that I blamed all sorts of people for causing me all sorts of problems. I did not see that the common factor in all my difficulties was me myself. Eventually, when my nearest and dearest told me that she, understandably, had had quite enough of me, I went to our doctor to ask what should be done about her and whether he felt there might be something that I might do that would be helpful to her. He, quite rightly, suggested that it was I who needed help. I remember thinking to myself that often in the course of my medical practice I make this same statement to patients and that on some occasions they respond by saying that the world looks sane enough to them. I tend to reply that their lives don't look quite so sane when seen from the outside. Faced with my own doctor saying the same thing to me, I accepted that I should "see" somebody.

But whom should I see? My GP did not think that he should take me on himself because he knew me too well personally. He therefore referred me to an analytical psychotherapist. In due course I lay on a couch, looked at the ceiling and the opposite wall, and went quietly mad. Without my normal handholds for emotional security, I fell apart. The psychotherapist therefore asked for "medical cover" and referred me to a very kind doctor who worked exclusively in the private sector as a general medical practitioner. He heard me through, patiently, and referred me to a consultant psychiatrist, who said to me, "I gather you want to break down". It struck me as an odd statement: "breaking down" was the last thing that I wanted to do. However, having placed myself in his hands I thought that I should follow his suggestions and therefore agreed to be admitted as an inpatient to a mental nursing home in north London. This was nowhere near my home area in Kensington and I felt very cut off. I was put into a side ward on my own, in a completely blank room with no pictures or ornaments of any kind. For three days I had no visitors whatever, not even the consultant psychiatrist himself, other than the ladies who brought me my meals. I had no contact with other patients - seventeen old ladies. My private medical insurance company were happy enough to pay the bill for the specialist, perhaps particularly when I decided that three days of total isolation was quite enough.

From that experience I learnt what I call "spiritual mathematics" $0 + 1 = 0$; $1 + 1 = 3$.

The explanation of these two equations is that by myself I get nowhere, whereas when I interact with other people, something extra comes into my life. That philosophy has stood me in good stead every since.

In due course when I went first to Overeaters Anonymous, then to Gamblers Anonymous and subsequently on to Addictions Anonymous, realising that I had more than just one addictive tendency. I learnt to become inter-dependent with other sufferers. I did not heal them and they did not heal me: we healed ourselves in the process of taking our minds off ourselves and putting them on to other people.

Subsequently as my interest and understanding increased, I undertook various professional psychotherapeutic training programmes: in Gestalt therapy, Transactional Analysis, Analytical Psychotherapy, Reality Therapy and Psychodrama - and on each occasion learnt a bit more about how disturbances of thought and feeling and behaviour can be helped. I went on these courses, not as a doctor but as myself. However, just as I had found many years previously when I had tried to sing professionally despite being medically qualified, other people find it very difficult to forget that I am a doctor. I suppose I look like a doctor and behave like one even when I am doing something completely different. However hard I may try to discard that role when singing or when attending a psychotherapy-training course, other people put it back on to me. This does not mean that they ask me questions about their medical ailments. It means that they have the image "doctor" so firmly printed in their minds that they are unable to see me in any other capacity. In my experience, this then causes them to be rather ill at ease. They see me as the cause of that nervousness and they react. Despite the fact that many singers earn their living as teachers, I was told firmly that I would never get anywhere as a singer unless I gave up being a doctor. There were other more fundamental reasons for my discontinuing my singing career - basically I wasn't good enough - but it was interesting to note that full-time teachers were none the less considered to be professional singers whereas I was seen as an amateur and a dilettante.

In some of the psychotherapy courses I was seen as "the enemy" - or at least that's how it appeared to me. I am not paranoid in other relationships in my life but, in the world of psychotherapy, doctors are not always perceived by patients as being their friends. Bearing in mind my own experience in the nursing home, I am not altogether surprised. Conversely, in the Anonymous Fellowships no one knows who I am - or they don't let on if they do. But in the psychotherapeutic world the label "doctor" tends to be stuck on my forehead - almost as a warning to those who might converse with me.

In one psychotherapeutic training course that disturbingly, and to my mind unhelpfully, involved beating cushions and screaming, it was suggested that I should beat a cushion labelled "mother". I responded that I had no intention whatever of doing that. I might at times want to beat a cushion labelled "mother's ideas" but otherwise I am at peace with my mother and have been for years as a result of working the Twelve Step Programme of the Anonymous Fellowships based upon principles first established by Alcoholics Anonymous. Another member of the psychotherapy group was then allowed to beat a cushion labelled "Robert" (me) and subsequently in another session, I was not formally de-roled after playing the part of an abusive parent in a role-play.

Do I ask for abuse or is it thrust upon me? Or am I simply too sensitive, relative to other people, when emotional abuse comes my way? How would I know? How could I judge from the inside? It is a commonplace that doctors find it difficult to ask for help. From my experience it is equally difficult to receive it when one does ask for it, particularly in the field of emotional health.

In the course of my life as a general medical practitioner I have had a number of other doctors as patients of mine and in the last fifteen years while running our addiction treatment centre, I have had twelve doctors as inpatients under my care. In each circumstance I try to remember that the patient just happens to be a doctor but that this is usually irrelevant to the condition that is being treated. The treatment for a sore throat or for diabetes or for drug addiction is exactly the same for doctors as it is for clergymen, politicians, students, or housewives. I might not necessarily have to explain a medical word or concept to another doctor - but generally I find it safer to act on the assumption that the doctor does not understand even medical words, let alone concepts. On the occasion when an ear, nose and throat surgeon looked at my larynx I was very glad that he explained things in simple terms: I did not want to have to rely upon my own medical knowledge of a subject in which he was the expert. Correspondingly, I have to assume that other doctors put themselves into my hands when they believe that I have some expertise as a general medical practitioner or as someone with significant experience of dealing with emotional problems and addictive or compulsive behaviour.

I suppose the guiding principles in trying to help one's own professional colleagues are firstly to recognise that it is an honour and privilege to do so and secondly to get on and treat them the same as one would treat anyone else. If helpers are to be helped ourselves, we need to be allowed to put aside that mantle for one brief moment so that we can be human, alongside everyone else.

Chapter Five

What is Help?

When John Collins prescribed two lots of tablets and an inhaler to deal with my chest infection due to mycoplasma, he doubled the number of tablets that I had taken in my entire life. I was so surprised to find that I needed anything at all. Normally when I get a cough or a cold I let it get better by itself in time but this particular cough had gone on for nearly a month. By and large I believe that the human body looks after itself very well and that the best thing we can do to help ourselves is to let nature take its course. However, on this occasion, that didn't work.

On a previous occasion when I caught Salmonella food poisoning from a chicken mayonnaise sandwich, I took no treatment - which is the correct thing to do for salmonella infections - and I was rid of the symptoms in less than a week. When John Stubbs took out my gallbladder - before the days of endoscopic (minimal access) surgery - I was up and about the day after the operation and then left hospital altogether two days later. In the days when I used to have toothache I treated it with oil of cloves. Occasional backache has been treated with physiotherapy. For all these various ailments I have been well served by the natural recuperative powers of my own body, aided on some occasions by specialist procedures, and there has been no need for "a pill for every ill". Obviously there are people who need regular medication for their ailments but, in general, I believe that doctors prescribe too much and patients take too much.

Even in preventive care we can become obsessed and either do or take too much. I don't take daily Aspirin to protect my heart and arteries because I have no significant cardiovascular risk: both of my parents lived into their nineties - my father is still alive at ninety-six - my blood pressure is at the level of a twenty year old, my cholesterol level likewise, and I do not smoke cigarettes, drink alcohol or caffeine, eat sugar or white flour or add salt. I don't believe in vitamin or trace element supplements: a healthy diet gives me all I need and supplements distort the natural balance. It may sound as if I have no fun in life but that is surely a reflection upon our culture in which things that are self-destructive have come to be considered to be a necessary part of life - and certainly more fun than things that are self-enhancing. However, I am aware that one does not cure an obsession for doing something by becoming obsessed over not doing it. Abstinence is the only effective treatment for addiction but we need to maintain a balance in all other areas of life. I suppose my greatest risks nowadays are from road accidents - as a result of driving when over-tired - or from being walloped for being insufferable.

In short, I try to live a healthy life and so far, by God's grace or by chance, I have been exceedingly fortunate. Far from being aware of what I have given up in the form of various addictive substances, I have almost boundless energy and a wide range of interests and activities, mainly in literature and the arts.

I believe that good health is largely a matter of attitude and of not doing things that are damaging. The best form of help that one can ever receive is not to need it in the first place. That principle works perfectly well for physical health, by and large, and maintenance of emotional health is similar. As body and mind work together, I believe that physical health in fact very much depends upon emotional health. My wife Meg and I worked through our earlier problems rather than ran away from them - and we find that there are very considerable benefits from having a long-term relationship. We understand each other and we enjoy each other's company. I have been exceedingly fortunate in my life in finding professional work that is so congenial to me. I have also been exceedingly fortunate in the privileges that life has brought me. To be sure I have earned them to some extent but I also have to acknowledge that I have been very lucky.

I have to some extent created that luck by taking advantage of my assets and not allowing my handicaps to dominate everything else. Apart from short sight and a severe allergy to bee stings, my only natural handicaps are those imposed upon me by my addictive tendency, which I believe is probably genetically inherited as it runs through all generations of my family in one way or another. Again, I have been exceedingly fortunate in having a chronic illness that is totally manageable on a day-to-day basis. It has devastating effects in some other people through their use of nicotine, alcohol, sugar and prescribed or recreational drugs but I have been totally relieved of my addictions by the continuing support that I receive in three meetings each week of various Anonymous Fellowships and by working the Twelve Step programme. This simple supportive and preventive measure leaves the rest of my life free for real enjoyment.

I do not believe that I have been healed of my basic addictive tendency. As with other addicts, it is still there as a potential for destruction every day of my life. But I am now free from compulsion and I am open-minded to new ideas in my personal and professional life. It is not simply a question of knowing that I would go crazy again if I were to relapse back to my former behaviour: it is more that I am aware of the incredible benefits that I get now each and every day. I can be myself rather than be driven by my compulsions. I have peace of mind in spite of unsolved problems. I have creativity, spontaneity and enthusiasm - features that make an incredible difference to the quality of my life.

Two further features - acceptance and gratitude - have transformed my actions and reactions. For example, Meg and I were obviously very sad when our lovely home was totally destroyed by an arsonist with whom we had no personal or professional connection whatever. But we survived and now we have an even prettier home. Three years after the event we are still fighting the insurance company but that's life - or, rather, that's insurance companies. This particular disaster was caused by someone else but, one way or another, I now recognise that I myself am the cause of most of my difficulties and I myself need to sort them out or come to terms with them.

Providing these extensive examples of my own attempts to maintain physical, emotional and mental health might be seen to be self-indulgent and self-satisfied. However, I write from personal experience and I tend to be unimpressed by people who write merely from theory or who say one thing but do another.

Thus, I believe that good physical and mental health is largely a matter of taking care of ourselves rather than being helped by other people. The helping professions would be largely unnecessary if patients looked after themselves better than they tend to do. Furthermore, the helping professions are not always as helpful as we might be because sometimes we create a dependency culture. We may even like it when people become dependent upon us because we believe that this gives our own professional lives - and even our personal lives - some validity. But this can be very damaging.

Compulsive helping, based upon the need to be needed, is widespread among the helping professions - and it is not an asset either to the patients or to the helpers. It can be very destructive indeed. This does not mean that compulsive helpers are incapable of altruism or of giving genuine help. However, it does mean that on some occasions the motivation for their actions will have more to do with their own psyche than to do with genuine observable benefit in the patient or other recipient. Compulsive helping is therefore invidious and although on many occasions it is trivial and inconsequential there are other times when it can be devastating.

Consider, for example, politicians who believe that their own vision of what is good for other people in social welfare cannot be challenged except by Nazis. Often at election times these politicians compete with each other to see who can give away even more of other people's money. Their policies can sometimes result in a dependency culture in which people make no attempt to improve their own condition but demand even more welfare services on the grounds of their "just deserts". Thus, the end result of the politicians' worthy care and concern is damaging to the creative sector of the economy, from which taxes are raised, and may also be damaging - through creating dependency - to those who receive state handouts.

As Ayn Rand pointed out, the difference between a Welfare State and a Totalitarian State is merely a matter of time. This is not to denigrate workers who give their best unstintingly in the service of their fellow men and women. It simply points out that we do not always get the results that we intend. Our efforts may contribute to other people's detriment rather than to their help. Nor does it imply that all politicians are totalitarian. It does however, confirm the belief of Dr William Glasser, the consultant psychiatrist author of "Choice Theory", that when someone says "I know what is good for you" we should run for our lives. It also confirms that we should examine our own actions to see if they provide genuine benefit rather than create even more dependency. If the need of the helper is to feel good about his or her own actions, almost regardless of observable results of giving this "help" to other people, then the process is a hindrance rather than a help.

For doctors, nurses and other health workers, the issue of compulsive helping is vitally important. Of course we should help our patients: that is what we are for. However, the yardstick should always be the question "Have my actions truly helped the patient?". We may believe that something should help - but does it? For example, we should question whether educating patients solely on the physical dangers of cigarette smoking does actually lead to them giving it up. Addicted smokers often know all about the risks of cigarette smoking and yet they still smoke. Giving information and advice to them is therefore both superfluous and patronising: it fails to diagnose the true nature of the problem, which is the addictive disease. Under such circumstances our real responsibility, in my view, is to find out how to deal with addiction in an effective manner rather than simply to repeat our previous advice and exhortations and continue with cognitive behavioural approaches that don't work for addicts. My emphasis on the benefits of a Twelve Step programme are not simply the result of my personal experience but because untreated addiction to alcohol, nicotine, sugar and recreational drugs is the cause of a simply vast number of medical conditions. Chronic bronchitis and emphysema, cancer of the lung and many other cancers, heart attacks, liver disease, obesity, accidents and suicide are all very considerably influenced by the use of addictive substances or behaviour. Furthermore, in contrast with expensive medical treatment after the event, the Twelve Step programme is preventive and free and therefore universally available.

When considering the plight of those less fortunate than ourselves, we should of course provide for those most in need. But where do we draw the line, how do we prevent the formation of a poverty trap, and how do we avoid leading patients into a dependency culture? The answer to these questions depends upon the courage of politicians, doctors and other health workers to say what we will *not* provide. The demand for health and welfare services is a bottomless pit that could easily absorb the entire gross national product of any country. Therefore there have to be limits to what is provided - and these limits are uncomfortable for politicians and for healthcare workers. We don't mind blaming each other for lack of funds or poor delivery of service but we are very reluctant to face an individual patient, or a group of patients or a pressure group, and say "I am not going to provide that service for you because the available resource is better spent in other ways on people whose need is greater" - but that is what we need to do. It values the resource.

Like it or not, health and welfare services are part of a general market, be it state or private. No budget is unlimited. Satisfying one demand simply switches the focus to another. We could in fact provide a National Health Service or set of charitable services on any budget whatever simply by specifying precisely what we are not prepared to pay for or provide. This may seem harsh - but reality is harsh. We cannot provide "health" to the nation because the concept of health is too nebulous. All we can do is to say what we will provide, and what we will not, within the budget at our disposal. Governments and healthcare providers could work together on this issue but generally we prefer to fight and blame each other for the inevitable failure to achieve Utopian expectations.

To be truly helpful to patients we need to start by being honest with them on what we can provide and what we can not. Furthermore, what we should focus upon most of all is to help patients to harness their own resources. As Professor Lawrence Weed of the University of Vermont emphasises, patients are the most valuable members of his "staff" because there is one to every patient and they are, most commonly, highly motivated to do whatever they can to help themselves when they can be shown how to do so. We tend to under-value this resource.

Furthermore, we may distance ourselves from our patients by becoming almost too scientific and not sufficiently human in our relationships with them, even while necessarily dressing ourselves in an appropriately smart, professional manner. Meeting their expectations of treatment or cure with the latest scientific wonders may not be possible either clinically or financially. Helping patients to understand and accept these limits is exceedingly difficult when healthcare workers collude with politicians and the press in raising people's expectations inappropriately. We need to explain that we do what we can within the limits of our resources and that sometimes we fail even under ideal circumstances. One problem may be solved only to reveal another and, ultimately through age and decay, we all die. This again is another harsh reality - and we have no choice but to face it and accept it.

When my mother was dying I asked that she should be left in peace in her nursing home. Instead I was told by the medical and nursing staff that they could not possibly do that: she deserved every opportunity to be restored to health. She was ninety-three years old, blind, almost deaf and generally incapacitated and in chronic pain. Pneumonia was her friend, not an enemy: it could have provided her a gentle and dignified death instead of the elaborate, painful and undignified performance that she endured in hospital with tubes stuck in her every orifice. Has it really come to this - that we have to brutalise old ladies because of our fear of being sued or being reported to our professional organisations or because of our need to "help"?

Chapter Six

Healing the Body

When asked the way to a particular village, an old man is said to have replied "Well ... I wouldn't start from here".

The same principle applies to healing one's own body: as far as possible we should avoid doing the things that cause us damage. Obviously, accidents will happen and all life involves some risk or other - but it is extraordinary how little care most of us give to our own bodies. Generally we know full well that we eat the wrong things and in the wrong quantities, that we may drink too much alcohol and that we should not smoke at all and certainly not use recreational drugs. We know that we should not take risks on the road, on or in the water, in high places or on building sites. We know that our own homes have risks of fire or falls, cuts, scalds, poisons or electrocution. We know the risks of bites or stings and other more serious accidents that can happen to us in our gardens or other places of recreation. We know the risks of various sporting activities such as boxing, rock climbing, horse riding and even basketball. We know the risks of getting into the wrong bed. Yet we take these risks - or at least some of them - because life without any risk at all would not be much fun for most of us, even if it were possible.

All that being said, however, we really don't need to go out of our way as far as we do to cause ourselves - and sometimes each other - avoidable harm.

I suppose it all depends upon what we want from life. For myself I want to be happy in my close personal relationships and I want to achieve something creative in my professional work. From that starting point I am aware that I am running out of time. I suppose theoretically I have always been running out of time from the moment I was born - but I am becoming more aware of it as I get older. It is improbable that I could now make a significant change in my career and I hope I never have to work on creating a second marriage. I therefore treasure what I have got and I try to avoid doing things that would jeopardise my health and happiness. On the other hand, all creative activity involves taking risks and all relationships have to grow if they are not to stagnate and regress. Inevitably things sometimes go wrong when we take risks - but hopefully we learn from our experience.

The body and mind work so closely together that it is impossible to separate physical, emotional and mental health. When we are physically healthy we feel good and we think clearly. When we are physically ill the opposite is the case. When we are emotionally or mentally disturbed we are more likely to become physically ill or to be involved in accidents. The whole physical, emotional and mental package acts as one and this totality could be termed our "spirit". If we respect our human spirit we will look after ourselves physically and emotionally and mentally, all with equal care, and we will get equal benefits.

Even so, sometimes we are just unlucky. We may have a genetic predisposition towards an illness or defect of some kind or other or we may develop an illness, or be involved in an accident, when we were really powerless to avoid it. One member of my close family has multiple congenital malformations and continues to have a whole series of operations and other treatments for various physical malfunctions and she requires many forms of educational and social support. Even her basic healing mechanisms do not work very well. She is more prone than other children to get ailments of one kind or another and she does not get over them as quickly as they do. There is nothing that she or anyone else can do about that: it is just the way that she is made.

For the rest of us, there is a great deal that we can do to influence our healing mechanisms but this involves putting significant effort into creating and maintaining physical, emotional and mental health. It does not simply come to us as a gift beyond our basic genetic inheritance. If we want good health, there is a great deal that we can do to create it - and we have to focus on all aspects of our lives. For example, it is pointless believing in "health foods" while continuing to smoke cigarettes. Equally, it is impossible to get emotional happiness and peace of mind simply as a result of working hard in a gymnasium. We may feel physically fitter but the quality of our relationships depends primarily upon our inter-actions with other people rather than what we do on our own. We may put ourselves in a good frame of mind through prayer and meditation but that won't help very much if at the same time we are dishonest and disrespectful. One way or another, the golden rule of "do as you would be done by" is the most significant of all stepping stones towards good health.

Focusing more specifically upon physical health, we would generally do well to let our bodies heal themselves as far as possible. If we have an ache or a pain it is best to investigate the cause rather than simply to treat the consequence. Taking painkillers may disguise the true nature of our problem. We need to ask for professional help if our symptoms do not resolve spontaneously in time. Usually we would tend to know perfectly well that we have a pain in the back because we lifted a heavy weight awkwardly or we have a sore throat because we caught the same germ that everybody else was getting at the same time, or we feel nauseous because of a bad meal. None of these things necessarily requires any investigation or treatment, although it would probably be sensible to ask for advice if the symptoms drag on for longer than a week. However, if we feel persistently unwell or if we have lost weight or if we have a pain that simply won't go away, then we should ask for help so that we can be diagnosed and treated before our illness, whatever it may be, becomes too advanced. We can do a great deal to help doctors and other professionals by being sensible in not asking for help over every little thing but in asking for it as early as possible when we really are worried about something. After all it is primarily the doctor's job, rather than the patient's, to decide - other than for trivial things - whether or not something really matters.

My own view from general medical practice is that my primary responsibility as a doctor is to listen, examine, investigate and diagnose rather than necessarily to treat. My consultations do not inevitably lead to a prescription. In many cases I don't trust pharmaceutical drugs to do what they purport to do without at the same time doing all sorts of other unwanted things. Anyway, I find that patients are often reassured when they know that they have been properly heard and examined. "Cook-book" medicine - giving a tablet for each and every symptom - is not responsible clinical practice, particularly with patients who are very young or very old because their bodies cannot cope with all these pharmaceutical substances. The drugs are not necessarily truly helpful anyway. Doctors take on a fearful responsibility when we become licensed to prescribe medicines. We should undertake that responsibility with care. It is small wonder that progressively more patients seek "alternative" remedies when they see how often we doctors reach for our prescription pads.

It is also true that surgeons may operate too readily. I remember Professor Harold Ellis at the Westminster Hospital giving a most illuminating talk on "Surgical retreats": operations that are no longer performed because they have been found to be unhelpful or even dangerous to the patients. There are wonderful things that surgeons can do but that does not necessarily mean that they should. For example, jaw-wiring operations, stomach stapling or intestinal shortening operations, all for the treatment of obesity, are attempts to treat an emotional problem - overeating - with a surgical treatment and that must be wrong. Similarly, heart transplant operations and coronary artery bypass operations should never be considered to be the appropriate treatment for the consequences of cigarette smoking: doctors attention should be focused primarily upon prevention rather than simply upon dramatic treatments. We doctors may like to consider that we are "doing" something - but we may not be doing the right thing at the right time.

That being said, the miracles of modern scientific medicine really are miracles - both medically and surgically. There is a very great deal that can be done and is being done to heal and save lives that would otherwise be chronically impaired or lost altogether. The "alternative" scene does not have all the answers - if any. It is indeed healthy to avoid taking a "pill for every ill" but it may be just as unhealthy to take a crack-pot remedy or to avoid getting an early diagnosis for a significant problem simply because one has a profound distrust of doctors. If people want to believe in "alternative" remedies then that is up to them - and I would share with them the belief that almost anything is often preferable to a pharmaceutical remedy. However, we should not lose sight of the basic scientific principle of being able to demonstrate in double blind controlled trials - in which neither the doctor nor the patient knows whether the treatment being prescribed is the genuine article or a placebo - that a specific treatment really does work and is not simply a branch of faith healing. I am all in favour of faith healing if the patient's symptoms are genuinely resolved but underlying disease processes must not be missed. Faith healers have their place - but so do doctors.

Chapter Seven

Healing the Mind

About one third of my work as a general practitioner involves dealing with emotional stresses of one kind or another and all my work in our addiction centre involves counselling. Generally I don't prescribe mood-altering drugs such as tranquillisers and anti-depressants. In my general medical practice I might occasionally give people a strip of ten sleeping tablets simply to break a cycle of insomnia but I would not normally prescribe them, or a tranquilliser or anti-depressant, for an acute emotional crisis, even after bereavement. I don't think they are necessary and I do think that they can get in the way of the body's natural healing processes. We may need to be able to grieve appropriately or work our way through the emotional challenges that life sends us. As I see it, my job is to ensure that there is no physical illness causing the emotional problem and then to provide appropriate support. On rare occasions I will refer for consultant psychiatric opinion if I believe that there may be specific mental illness. Out of a total of six thousand consultations each year, I might refer three or four patients for a psychiatric opinion. I might prescribe sleeping tablets about once a week and tranquillisers and anti-depressants only if I am continuing another doctor's prescription while the patient transiently passes through London.

I don't believe that my patients are particularly healthy or unhealthy. I see the same patients - or their equivalents - as other doctors in my geographical area. I have worked in South Kensington for twelve years in the National Health Service and subsequently in fully private practice. I did not prescribe mood-altering drugs any more frequently when I worked in the NHS practice than I do now. I am exceedingly familiar with the stresses and strains of living in a city centre and I am just as familiar with the emotional and social problems of those who are underprivileged as I am with those who have considerable privilege. None of these patients necessarily needs psychoactive pharmaceutical substances. They don't need pills to make them feel better. They need a bit of care and a bit of time.

Some doctors argue that they don't have time to treat emotional problems and that they cannot resolve the social issues that might be the underlying cause and therefore they have no choice but to prescribe. I fundamentally disagree. There is always time in general medical practice to do whatever one wants to do: it is all a matter of organisation and appropriate delegation.

When I was still working in the National Health Service, I decided to spend money on having pleasant premises for my professional work. After all, I spend most of my life in them and only a relatively short time at home. Equally, I decided to employ good staff and pay them well. I still do. As a result, my staff tends to stay with me for many years. Thus, the basics of my professional life are very stable even though the local population - in bed-sit land - has a high social morbidity and high turnover rate. I see a wide variety of clinical and social problems every day of my life and about one in five of my consultations each day is on a patient I have never seen before. No one can question the demands upon me and upon the population that I serve - yet still I do not prescribe and still I find the time to deal with patient's emotional problems. The solution is in having long consultation hours, efficient management by the staff, and effective delegation of clinical problems that I do not believe require my professional skills, such as they may be. In other words, the solutions are primarily those of management and motivation. Neither of these subjects are taught in medical school - and I doubt whether they can be: you either have the talent for them or you don't. My concern again is that people may be inadequately selected - if at all - for a career in general medical practice. We enter it armed with our knowledge of treatment for diseases of the body and yet largely on a day-to-day basis, we treat dis-eases of the mind and spirit.

In my work in the addiction field, on an outpatient basis in London during the week and on an inpatient basis in Kent at the weekends, my work is exclusively in counselling. I delegate all medical problems to other doctors whom I employ. I do this because I do not wish this particular group of patients to be able to see me in any other capacity than as the head of the counselling team. There is no point in them trying to wheedle drugs out of me because I simply do not prescribe drugs other than for the "detoxification" processes for the first few days of treatment. My prime function is to help patients to acknowledge that their difficulties are largely self-created, over and above their genetically inherited addictive nature. Correspondingly, I train the counselling staff and the nursing staff to do less rather than more for the patients than their natural instincts might lead them to do. Patients learn best when they work through their problems rather than have them solved by other people. They need the support and challenge of other patients in the group but they do not need counselling staff to tell them what to do. Our job as counsellors is to facilitate the processes of learning. We structure the day and we supervise the group processes, we provide insights from our experience but, by and large, we do not do things *for* patients: we help them to learn how to do things for themselves.

The great tragedy of clinical practice in our time is the over-prescription of mood-altering drugs such as tranquillisers, anti-depressants and sleeping tablets. These drugs never truly help anybody: they simply stick a plaster on the underlying wound but do nothing for the wound itself. A survey done by Professor Geoffrey Stephenson, Emeritus Professor of Psychology at the University of Kent at Canterbury, who heads our research department, showed that our patients in the addiction recovery centre have a higher general psychiatric morbidity than those in general psychiatric in-patient wards. In other words, we are looking after a more disturbed population. Yet still we do not prescribe drugs except for detoxification or for episodes of acute psychosis. I believe that patients with schizophrenia or manic depression require anti-psychotic or mood-stabilising medications - but I want to be absolutely sure of the diagnosis in the first place. Often we see patients who have been diagnosed as having schizophrenia when in fact their disordered thought processes were drug-induced. Equally we have seen many patients whose alcoholism was mis-diagnosed as manic depression.

The over-diagnosis and mis-diagnosis of depression is of particular concern. People who are depressed may in fact be suffering from the inner emptiness that is characteristic of an addictive tendency. Thus depression and addiction are, in my view, the same process, before and after "treatment" with a drug. Sadness, the emotional response to upsetting circumstances, is a separate clinical condition that requires no treatment at all other than emotional support, understanding and time. Anti-depressants, I believe, work on exactly the same principle that heroin works for toothache: they may take away the symptoms but they do nothing whatever for the underlying problem. I do not believe that antidepressants help patients to see the world and their problems more clearly. I believe that patients taking anti-depressants become imprisoned in a narrow band of emotional experience, feeling neither the highs nor the lows. This is a terrible thing to do to people. One would have hoped that Aldous Huxley's "*Brave New World*" would have shown that the way to spiritual hell is paved with prescription medications - but obviously not. Huxley's "Soma" is with us now - and it is called Prozac or Seroxat or Lustral or the name of any of the other selective serotonin re-uptake inhibitors, the "wonder drugs" of the moment.

We baffle ourselves with the science of brain biochemistry. We listen in admiration as specialists rattle off the beneficial effects and side effects of various psychoactive drugs, but even their knowledge is infinitesimal in the amazing complexity of brain function. Yet even that is not my major point - which is that we do not need to prescribe and we should not prescribe if there are alternative effective treatments.

Where problems are socially induced then the solutions need to be focused upon changing the aspects of society that are causing the problem. Where problems are domestic in origin then the focus should be upon the inter-relationships and other features of the domestic environment that may be the cause of the difficulty. In neither case - social or domestic - could medications remotely possibly have a place in treatment. We don't mend holes in the road with tablets and we should not attempt to mend the damage to people's minds or spirits with medications until the human brain has been given a chance to mend itself - as it frequently does. Getting people off psychoactive medications is often the most important first step in this process.

The brain has powers of recuperation that are just as remarkable as those of any other part of the body. In this sense the brain is very unlike a computer. Thinking of the brain as a computer belittles it, even taking into account some of the remarkable functions of modern computers. The brain's capacity for continuing to function despite severe disruption to a part of its physical structure, is truly amazing. Its capacity to select what it will remember is incredibly valuable: it scans and then chooses what it values for long-term memory. Its capacity to differentiate between thought and feeling can at times be problematic but for the most part this facility serves us well: we can still function and often work our way out of difficult situations even when we are emotionally distraught. Even the extreme circumstance of post-traumatic stress disorder can nowadays be helped through the therapeutic process of EMDR (eye movement desensitization and re-processing) in which the brain's natural recuperative powers are re-harnessed.

Psychotherapeutic processes have moved on a great deal - or should have done - in the last hundred years. What Freud began, others have continued - sometimes without making any progress whatever - but, for the most part, ideas have developed and new therapeutic approaches provide far more understanding and healing than classical analytical psychotherapeutic approaches ever achieved. There is a bizarre feature of the interaction between some therapists and patients in which it is sometimes believed that anything that is therapeutic has to be complicated. This idea dies hard. Both analysts and their patients may grind away interminably, with little evidence of clinical improvement. Yet even in Freud's own lifetime other, to my mind greater, therapists were showing a new way. Jacob Levy Moreno, the originator of psychodrama said "Dr Freud, you analysed their dreams; I try to give them courage to dream again".

Fritz Perls, the originator of Gestalt Therapy and Eric Berne, the originator of Transactional Analysis took up the challenge that Moreno had established in treating patients' thoughts, feelings and behaviours all at the same time. Cognitive Behavioural approaches and the "Rational Emotive Behaviour Therapy" of Albert Ellis have both sometimes set back that process by encouraging therapists to outwit or browbeat their patients, but Dr William Glasser's "Choice Theory" has restored humanity to the consultation and therapeutic process.

Neuro-Linguistic Programming was in vogue for a time and certainly has a point when it encourages us to examine the words that we use, particularly in the messages that we give to ourselves. Cognitive Analytical Therapy attempts to bring classical psychotherapeutic approaches to the aid of a wider population by making them more prescriptive - establishing particular frameworks and procedures - and reducing the timescale of the inter-action between therapist and patient. Whether it works any better than the full drawn-out version is debatable. Carl Rogers, through "person-centred" counselling turns the consultation process on its head and endeavours to see the patient's predicament primarily from his or her own perspectives rather than from those of the therapist. All these and many other psychological approaches continue to develop, as does the pharmaceutical industry's pursuit of "magic bullets". It is almost a race to the death: some therapists may try to encourage patients to come off medication while some doctors search for even more opportunities to prescribe.

A truly remarkable discovery was made by Dr Francine Shapiro in California in 1987. She discovered that the simple process of moving one's eyes repeatedly from one side to the other had a beneficial effect on the emotionally traumatic associations of images, physical sensations, emotional feelings and negative self-beliefs that might be the focus of one's attention at that particular time. Subsequent SPECT scans have shown that any alternating stimulation of both sides of the body result in the left (thinking) side of the brain being activated at the same time as the right (feeling) side of the brain. Thus, post-traumatic stress disorder, phobias and other clinical conditions originating many years previously and remaining stuck in the emotional memories of the right side of the brain, become accessible to the considered assessment of the left side of the brain whereas previously they had mostly been shut out. More recent traumas may also be processed so that the adaptive powers of the brain can be harnessed before these experiences become walled off as foci for post-traumatic stress disorder. At last a simple physiological technique, in trained professional hands, has been developed to enable thoughts to deal with feelings. It all sounds too good to be true but there is very considerable research evidence on controlled trials that support Dr Shapiro's ideas. In contrast, there are virtually no controlled trials supporting other therapeutic approaches, many of which simply rely upon the combined fervent belief of therapist and patient that so much investment of time and money must surely achieve something positive. EMDR, in skilled and properly trained hands, is effective and quick and is a highly refreshing antidote to the hocus pocus that surrounds a great deal of psychotherapy. EMDR can also reduce the perceived need in the minds of doctors and patients for psychoactive medications to be prescribed and that must surely be good. Jung, Moreno, Perls, Berne and Glasser have a worthy, humane, successor in Francine Shapiro.

Chapter Eight

Healing Relationships

Twenty years after the event I tried to make amends to one of my university contemporaries for my behaviour towards him at the time that we were undergraduates together. He turned round and walked away - and he had every right to do that. He did not want anything more to do with me. I had damaged the relationship irretrievably. Unfortunately, those of us who are addicts often do that. In the full flowering of our addictive disease we are so self-centred and tied up with our own issues, blaming others and pitying ourselves, that we leave a trail of destruction behind us. The fact that I am an addict does not excuse in any way the damage that I did to other people. I am totally responsible for my behaviour towards other people, always have been and always will be.

At the time of my disgraceful behaviour towards my contemporary, I was oblivious to my own responsibility. I blamed everyone else except myself. I blamed my family, my school, other students, the university and, most of all, the Government. Nothing and nobody was good enough for me. I was the only one who understood my pain and what I really needed. I lived in a world of emotional isolation even while surrounded by friends who, because I selected them, mostly lived in similar worlds to mine.

It was impossible at that time to get through to me. I was so self-obsessed that there was no chance of anybody else making a reasonable relationship with me. I emphasise this because sometimes a relationship may break down for entirely understandable reasons: one person may simply destroy it and there is nothing that the other person can do. Compulsive helpers sometimes stay in abusive relationships because they believe that there is something that they can do, particularly if they change their own behaviour in some way. This is an equivalent sickness or "co-dependency" - the only time I ever use that word which has come to mean so many different things that it really means nothing at all unless clearly defined as in this case.

Outside that particular circumstance - which is distressingly common, because addictive disease probably affects ten per cent of the population and therefore a considerable number of relationships - one should be able to get along with most people and even form close personal relationships with them.

Now that I am in recovery on a day-to-day basis from my addictive disease I have a wide range of friends. With some of my closest friends I have very little in common socially or professionally but we just seem to get along. We like each other and we respect our differences. However, I suspect that we would get on well even if we lived or worked together more closely. One reason for that is that I simply don't have the enemies that I used to have. I see people as friends until proven otherwise and that proof never seems to come.

Bureaucrats try my patience but even that is probably more of a reflection of my own wish to have everything finished by yesterday - and bureaucracy does not work that way because it has to make sure that everything is done in the right way. There are times when I get exasperated by this process - and say so - but nonetheless I do not personalise it: I am usually irritated by the process rather than by individual people.

Of course there are people with whom I have no wish to socialise and no desire to create any personal or professional relationship. I choose to have neither a personal nor a professional relationship with them. Why should I do otherwise?

Closer to home, my brother and I are different and we respect those differences. Politically and philosophically we are miles apart but I do not see that this should affect our personal relationship. We can afford to agree to differ. Among my friends I tend to be more at home with musicians, actors and artists than I am with doctors, but this simply reflects the first loves of my life rather than having anything specifically to do with the people themselves.

I believe that, except in the previous extreme circumstances such as I have described, I should be able to make a friendly relationship with almost anyone. The techniques of doing so are not exactly rocket science: simple consideration and good manners are about all there is to it. I have had a lot of experience of healing relationships because I have damaged so many in the past. I found that mostly what I needed to do to heal these relationships was to change my own behaviour irrespective of the other person's. Once I took responsibility for my own reactions as well as my actions, then my relationships steadily improved. What matters to me nowadays is the sharing of values on principles, ideas, interpretations and instincts. I find that this gives me a very broad range of friendships. I may share a particular feature with someone and value that so highly that I don't really notice other differences.

Equally, I have learnt to accept responsibility for my feelings as well as for my thoughts. I now believe that feelings are a direct reflection of whether my actions match my values. I feel bad when I know perfectly well that I am doing something that is in conflict with my values and I feel good when they are in agreement. I am at liberty to change either my actions or my values but I cannot complain if they are not in tune with each other: I therefore have only myself to blame for how I feel.

Harbouring resentments has been a particularly destructive feature of my life, as is common among addicts. My headmaster at school told me that he would not let me study music because "music is for homosexuals and we don't have that sort of thing here". I carried that resentment for twenty-five years until I recognised that the man obviously had a problem of some kind either with music or with homosexuality but there was no reason why I should continue to let that affect me. He lived in my head for too long. Nowadays I find it easier to avoid letting resentments build up in the first place.

I use myself as an example in illustrating the points I make because I do not feel that I have the ability to observe other people's motives. In working a Twelve Step programme on a day-to-day basis I have spent a long time digging out my own craziness and trying to put something better in its place. I have had so much work to do on myself that I have had little time or inclination to try to correct other people's behaviour. Inevitably my relationships have benefited from that: people tend to prefer it when I make no attempt to change them but simply accept them as they are. I do not have to accept their behaviour if it hurts me but I do not feel the need to preach to them or lecture them. My life is much more peaceful now that I no longer have a crusade to change everyone else. I work to change ideas, attitudes and opinions but I accept that other people have an equal right to challenge my own ideas, attitudes and opinions. It has to be a two-way process, or at least have the prospect of being so, if there is to be any development in the relationship or even in the ideas, attitudes and opinions themselves.

I believe that when relationships break down it happens most commonly because one person has been trying to change the other, or perhaps because they have both been trying to change each other. The strain is simply too great. Anger quickly boils into resentment. Understanding, acceptance and forgiveness go out of the window when the focus is all the time upon what the other person has done wrong. The only person one can ever change is oneself and acceptance of that fact is the beginning and end of healing one's own relationships.

Healing other people's relationships is a daunting task, yet that is what one attempts to do in counselling. I believe the secret of success is to focus upon the individuals, helping each to establish his or her own identity and values. After that they can decide for themselves what form they wish their relationship to take. On this principle, I do not see it as a failure of my own clinical skill when the relationship between two other people breaks down despite the help that I may have been giving them. On the same basis I give myself no credit when other people's relationships are healed. I might be the catalyst but I am not the instrument: they themselves are the instrument. I might take some credit for whatever skills I may have in my professional work as a counsellor in helping people to understand themselves and each other but I take no credit nor blame for the outcome in their particular relationship with each other. Perhaps it was best for that relationship to fold. How would I know? I have difficulty enough in monitoring my own relationships without presuming that I can interpret relationships between two other people in anything other than general psychological terms.

Sometimes people expect me as a counsellor to wave a magic wand. That cannot happen. Each of us is totally responsible for our own relationships and there is no magic wand that anyone else can wave.

My wife and I have been through many of the challenges that married couples face but, by and large, we have been very fortunate. Four things we have mercifully not experienced are the death of a child, chronic physical illness, poverty and unemployment. I cannot be sure that we would survive the pressures of those circumstances but I am sure that we would give it a try - and that surely is what it is all about. Running away from difficulties is easy: anyone can do that. Working through the challenges that life throws at us is what really makes the difference between those relationships that survive and those that falter. It is far more productive to focus upon what the other person says about our behaviour than upon how we ourselves justify it. It is far more constructive to let go of resentments, however much they may be justified, than to count them on a continuing basis. If we cannot let go then there is not much point in going on - but we shall have only ourselves to blame if we find that we repeat exactly that same process in the next relationship that we make.

Recently I have been trying to help a young girl who has had an addictive relationship with alcohol and drugs. We got her off all these substances and we were beginning to help her to see that a lot of her complaints about her family were because she saw them through the murky haze of her own addiction. Unfortunately, her mother reacted very strongly to the concept that her daughter might be an addict and therefore had her transferred to a psychiatric hospital where she was given "real" treatment - with drugs. Obviously I have my opinions about the relationship between the mother and daughter - but there is nothing that I can actually do about it. Also I have my opinions about the doctor who put the girl back onto mood-altering drugs, albeit prescription medications, when we had so carefully withdrawn drugs from her - but there is nothing I can do about that either. I cannot now have a professional relationship with the girl because she is under the care of another doctor. I cannot have a professional relationship with the mother because she absolutely does not want it - and I have to accept that as well. Both personal and professional relationships can be difficult at times. That is just the way it is. All that any one of us can do is simply to focus upon our own behaviour and let go of how other people behave towards us. In this particular girl's case I need to examine whether my own diagnosis and management were correct and whether I did the best I possibly could for her. There is nothing to be gained now by my focusing upon the behaviour of anyone else involved in this saga. I cannot learn from their experience: I can learn only from my own.

Other books in the series